HOW TO GAIN MORE INCHES

A Visual Manual on How to Increase Your Penis Size Naturally From The Comfort Of Your Bedroom

Included: Untold Secrets Of Adding More Inches

FRED JOEL

Copyright©2018

COPYRIGHT

TABLE OF CONTENT

CHAPTER 1 ....**4**

INTRODUCTION 4

CHAPTER 2 ....**6**

EIGHT WAY APPROACH TO INCREASE THE SIZE 6

CHAPTER 3STYLE **40**

ADDITIONAL TIPS 40

CHAPTER 4 ....**67**

DIET TO ACHIEVE A HEATHY PENIS 67

CHAPTER 5 ....**72**

UNTOLD SECRETS OF ADDING MORE INCHES 72

THE END **82**

CHAPTER 1

INTRODUCTION

Do you think that having a larger penis will lead to a better intercourse existence and extra self belief? I say HELL YEAH, you're totally right!

Read carefully, because you will find out a number of the pleasant sporting activities so that it will make your erections larger, stronger and extra satisfying. Simple as that!

Don't waste your precious time and money on merchandise that aren't going to do a unmarried factor. At the very worst, cheap tablets and gadgets can damage your health.

So what's the solution then? Are there any powerful ways to grow your dick that surely work? YUP – there are. The exceptional component is that you could do them at domestic with your arms handiest.

At the quit of this workout, you may get the great length of dick you seek for.

CHAPTER 2

EIGHT WAY APPROACH TO INCREASE THE SIZE

#1. ULTIMATE STRETCHER

Step #1:

a) Right after the warm-up phase, retract your foreskin & grasp your penis right behind its head (glans) firmly.

b) Pay attention not to cut off too much blood circulation (you should not feel any discomfort).

TheStallionStyle.com

EXTRA TIPS

This is a perfect workout for growing length

two You will want to attain between 0-30% erection

Take brief breaks between each stretch if necessary

Repeat this method 2 instances in every direction

Your session should last for 5-10 minutes

Improves: Length

Difficulty level: Beginner

Risk of injury: Small

Time required: 5-10 Minutes

The "ULTIMATE STRETCH" is amazing method specifically for these who want to enhance their length. It is a easy tactic that entails just stretching your flaccid little chum out.

Here are certain directions:

1. Take your time for a ideal warm-up phase.

2. Retract your foreskin and draw close your phallus at the back of (about one inch below) its head/glans firmly.

3. You have to experience no pain or large discomfort (do now not cut off too plenty blood circulation).

4. Pull it outwards with ample pressure to feel painless stretch inside your shaft.

5. Hold that position for 20 to 30 seconds.

6. If needed, rest for 5 seconds.

7. Repeat steps 2 to 4 but this time pull it upwards to your belly button.

8. Repeat but this time pull it downwards to your knees.

Fred Joel

9. Repeat however this time pull it to your right side.

10. Repeat but this time pull it to your left side.

11. Take your time to go through a cool down phase.

#2. THUMB STRETCHER

Step #1:

c) Pull & stretch your penis outwards in front of you.

a) Right after the warm-up phase, retract your foreskin & grasp your penis right behind its head (glans) firmly.

b) Pay attention not to cut off too much blood circulation (you should not feel any discomfort).

TheStallionStyle.com

EXTRA TIPS:

Ideal method for gaining length

Achieve between 0-30% erection

Alternate spots the place you area your thumb to unfold features evenly

One session need to last for 2-3 minutes

Improves: Length

Difficulty level: Advanced

Risk of injury: Medium

Time required: 2-3 Minutes

The "THUMB STRETCHER" is a barely one-of-a-kind technique you must add to your size boosting regime as well:

1. Take your time for a proper warm-up phase.

2. Retract your foreskin and hold close your phallus at the back of (about one inch below) its head/glans firmly.

3. You pull it outwards besides feeling any pain or good sized discomfort.

4. Use your other hand to place a thumb at the base of your penis (first third).

5. Press with your thumb down in the course of your knees.

6. You need to pull in each instructions at the same time with sufficient force to experience a painless stretch inside your shaft.

7. Hold that position for 20 to 30 seconds.

8. If needed, rest for 5 seconds between every repetition.

9. Repeat steps 2-7 4 instances in one session but alternate the spot where you vicinity your thumb.

10. Take your time to go via a cool down phase.

#3. BACKWARD PULLER

Step #1:

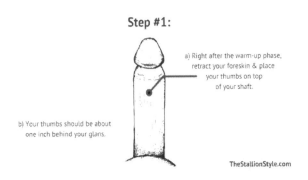

a) Right after the warm-up phase, retract your foreskin & place your thumbs on top of your shaft.

b) Your thumbs should be about one inch behind your glans.

TheStallionStyle.com

EXTRA TIPS:

Achieve between 30-75% erection

Alternate spots where you place your thumb to spread features evenly

Your session need to last for 4-6 minutes

Improves: Length & skin

Difficulty level: Beginner

Risk of injury: Medium

Time required: 4-6 Minutes

All you want to do in the BACKWARD PULLER is to comply with these steps:

1.   Take your time for a desirable warm-up phase.

2.   Retract your foreskin and region your thumbs on the pinnacle of your shaft one inch at the back of its head/glans.

3.   Place different fingers on each palms on the bottom facet of your shaft to support it.

4.   Pull the skin on top of your penis with your thumbs in the course of your body.

5.   Use sufficient force to feel a painless stretch and anxiety in your shaft.

6.   Hold that function for about 15-25 seconds.

7.   If needed, relaxation for 5 seconds between each repetition.

8.   Repeat steps 2-7 ten instances in one session however trade the spot the place you location your thumbs.

9.   Take your time to go thru a cool down phase.

While this exercising is now not that fantastic per se, it is a awesome addition to your PE pursuits and offers a little different type of tension for your penis.

#4. OPPOSITE STRETCH

Step #1:

a) Right after the warm-up phase, retract your foreskin & grasp your penis right behind its head (glans) firmly.

c) Pull & stretch your penis outwards in front of you (you should feel no pain).

b) Pay attention not to cut off too much blood circulation (you should not feel any discomfort).

TheStallionStyle.com

EXTRA TIPS:

Ideal for gaining length

Achieve between 0-30% erection

Begin with 6 repetitions

Your session have to ultimate for 3-5 minutes

Improves: Length

Difficulty level: Beginner

Risk of injury: Low

Time required: 3-5 Minutes

The OPPOSITE STRETCH is an exercise that would possibly make you flinch a little simply reading about it! However, make no mistake, as it's very nice and will expand your size, specifically length.

All you need to do is just comply with 9 simple steps:

1.   Take your time for a proper warm-up phase.

2.   Retract your foreskin and grasp your phallus at the back of (about one inch below) its head/glans firmly.

3.   You should feel no ache or giant soreness (do not reduce off too a whole lot blood circulation).

4.   With your second hand, grip the shaft with a popular ok-grip (between thumb and index finger) an inch above the base.

5.   Pull your first hand upwards away from and your 2nd hand downwards to your base with adequate pressure to sense painless stretch inner your shaft.

6.   Hold that function for 20 to 30 seconds.

Fred Joel

7.   If needed, rest for 5 seconds.

8.   Repeat steps 2 to 7 until you reach a preferred wide variety of repetitions.

9.   Take your time to go through a cool down phase

#5. KEGELS

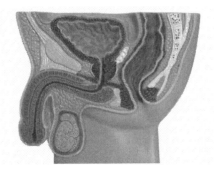

EXTRA TIPS:

Ideal for enhancing the great of your erections

Vary between brief soft and lengthy strong flexes

Gradually increase a number of and subject of flexes

You can do this kind of exercising anytime

Your session have to remaining at least 20-30 minutes

Improves: Erection

Difficulty level: Beginner

Risk of injury: Low

Time required: 20-30 Minutes

It's frequent expertise that Kegel workouts are really useful to women´s fitness in a variety of ways. However, very few men know that you can considerably enhance the blood drift and pleasant of your erections.

Your dick will appear large simply with the aid of preserving more manage over the erection itself! All you need to do is the following:

1.   Identify your Pubococcygeus (PC) muscle by using making an attempt a method of stopping your urine waft naturally.

2.   Once located, you will want to contract the PC muscle.

3.   Hold this contraction for at least 5 seconds.

4.   Release and take a spoil for 2 seconds.

5.   Repeat steps 2-4 till you end the preferred quantity of repetitions.

6.   Your each day session closing for 20-30 minutes.

Once you master these, you need to go for more contractions per day and session. Eventually, you'll be able to now not solely feel, but to control the muscle itself! There are a variety of regimes you may want to strive out.

This workout will lead to a substantial enhance in quality of your erections as extra blood will waft to your dick. Trust me that your woman will be conscious of your positive aspects and your rock-hard boners!

#6 - WET JELQING

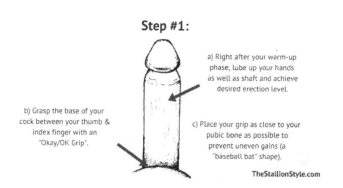

Step #1:

a) Right after your warm-up phase, lube up your hands as well as shaft and achieve desired erection level.

b) Grasp the base of your cock between your thumb & index finger with an "Okay/OK Grip".

c) Place your grip as close to your pubic bone as possible to prevent uneven gains (a "baseball bat" shape).

TheStallionStyle.com

EXTRA TIPS:

Achieve between 50-75% erection

Never jelq your glans

Start with small wide variety of repetitions (20)

Gradually amplify the wide variety of repetitions per session

Stop as quickly as you begin to sense any discomfort

Improves: Girth & length

Difficulty level: Beginner

Risk of injury: Low

Time required: 1+ Minutes

Before beginning with the jelqing exercise make certain that you're already at least semi-erect (between ½ and ¾ of your maximum erection power).

Now you have to follow these steps:

1.   Take your time for a applicable warm-up phase.

2.   Lubricate each your palms and your shaft well (use oil based totally lube).

3.   Achieve desired erection level.

4.   With your right hand hold close the base of your cock between your thumb and index finger with an "OK/OKAY GRIP".

5.   Place your grip as close to your pubic bone as feasible to avoid uneven positive aspects (baseball bat shape).

6.   Tighten your grip so you will painlessly trap the blood in your shaft.

7.   Slowly slide your hand (it need to take you 2-3 seconds) up to the glans and practice sufficient stress with your grip to force blood up your penis.

8. Stop sliding your hand simply before it reaches your glans (at this point you have finished one jelq).

9. While nonetheless keeping your one hand right before your glans, use your different hand to "OKAY GRIP" the base of your cock.

10. Again area your grip as close to your pubic bone as possible.

11. Release your first hand that is gripping right before your glans.

12. Return to the step #6 and proceed until you attain the favored variety of repetitions.

13. Do no longer forget to take your time to go through a cool down phase.

As a beginner, think about a decrease range of repetitions per single session and then extend this quantity gradually. If you want extra precise information, then take a look at out my latest article to analyze how to make your penis higher with jelqing technique.

PAY ATTENTION:

Jelqing your glans can also result in loss of its sensitivity

Jelqing with a flaccid cock will gain no gains

Jelqing with a one hundred percent erection may often end result in a soft tissue & nerve damage

#7. ROTATING STRETCH

Step #1:

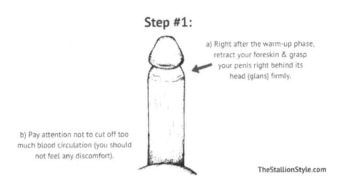

a) Right after the warm-up phase, retract your foreskin & grasp your penis right behind its head (glans) firmly.

b) Pay attention not to cut off too much blood circulation (you should not feel any discomfort).

TheStallionStyle.com

EXTRA TIPS:

Ideal approach for gaining length

Achieve between 0-30% erection

Stretch for 20-30 seconds in each course (clockwise & counterclockwise)

Your session have to closing for 2-3 minutes

Improves: Length

Difficulty level: Beginner

Risk of injury: Low

Time required: 3+ Minutes

This approach is very similar to the first exercising on this list. However, there are some differences you want to pay interest to.

You will want to observe these steps:

1.   Take your time for a suitable warm-up phase.

2.   Retract your foreskin and grasp your phallus with and "OKAY GRIP" in the back of (about one inch below) its head/glans firmly.

3.   Pull it outwards with ample force to trip a painless stretch interior your shaft.

4.   While keeping your grip and stretch, you need to go your penis in a circular motion.

5.   When gripping with your proper hand, commence your circle to the left and proceed counterclockwise.

6.   When gripping with your left hand, start your circle to the right and proceed clockwise.

7.   When stretching downwards, preserve your hand as shut to your physique as possible.

8.   One rotation should ultimate for 20-30 seconds.

9. You can swap your palms after ending your rotation as needed.

10. Repeat steps 2-9 and rotate at least 3 instances in every direction.

11. Take your time to go thru a cool down phase.

Don't continue if you experience any pain or discomfort. All these workout routines were designed to be pain-free.

#8. WEIGHT-LIFTER

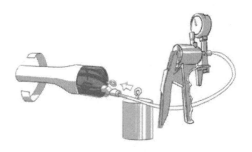

EXTRA TIPS:

Penis hangers come with protection risks (do your research first)

Rather choose a vacuum-based system as it does no longer block blood circulation

You should amplify the weight gradually

Penis hangers and weights have been popularized over the years by using Japanese, and have indeed been proven to work on various occasions. The exceptional option is a vacuum-based device, such as "LG Hanger", but you can try a constriction-based choice (more dangerous) such as "Bib Hanger" or "Zen Hanger" as well.

Here are 4 steps that you will want to follow with weight hanging:

1.   Always attempt this technique on your flaccid "manhood".

2.   Attach a unique weight to your hanger that has been created solely for this purpose.

3.   This will force it to stretch downwards like in other strategies mentioned right here already.

4.   Doing this must make your dick measurement larger steadily – in a permanent way.

You have to consider doing a little greater research before attempting this as it's probably very harmful!

CHAPTER 3

ADDITIONAL TIPS

IMPROVE BLOODFLOW WITH MALE EXTRA PILLS

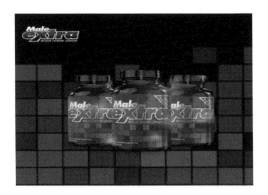

While doing workout routines above will supply you with excellent results, you can improve your success fee by way of enhancing the blood waft into your penis. Male Extra is one of the most promising enhancement capsules on the market (even provides an fine money-back guarantee).

This brand claims to beautify your sex life by:

• Improving your libido and stamina

• Forcing tougher and extra excessive erections

- Permanent increase of your size

The consequences aren't seen overnight, but you will see boom in 3 to 6 months. Anyone struggling from a smaller penis or any individual who just desires to achieve a bigger, tougher erection is aware of that three months are nothing if you can obtain 0.8 to 2.6 inches.

#2. TRY WATER BASED PENIS PUMP

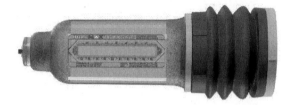

Using penis pumps is a GREAT WAY to expand your size. By pumping, you will create a suction that will increase the blood drift to your penis, growing a very sturdy and massive erection. This way, it makes a outstanding addition to your penis growth routine.

I have a personal advice for you.

Instead of usual vacuum pumps (these are greater dangerous) use rather hydro-based suction pumps as these are safer and much extra effective.

There are two most dependable manufacturers on the market right now:

– Bathmate (better product)

– Penomet

These two are fantastic merchandise that have a water chamber allowing for a very blissful use. Although your outcomes will be solely brief in the beginning, with the right events you can cement beneficial properties you will achieve with above exercises.

#3. USE RELIABLE PENIS EXTENDER

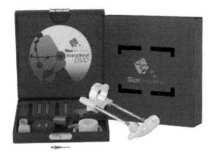

Using penis pumps is a GREAT WAY to expand your size. By pumping, you will create a suction that will increase the blood drift to your penis, growing a very sturdy and massive erection. This way, it makes a outstanding addition to your penis growth routine.

I have a personal advice for you.

Instead of usual vacuum pumps (these are greater dangerous) use rather hydro-based suction pumps as these are safer and much extra effective.

There are two most dependable manufacturers on the market right now:

– Bathmate (better product)

– Penomet

These two are fantastic merchandise that have a water chamber allowing for a very blissful use. Although your outcomes will be solely brief in the beginning, with the right events you can cement beneficial properties you will achieve with above exercises.

#4. USE LUBES WITH NUTRITIONAL SUPPORT

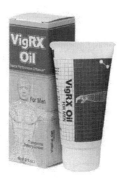

Thanks to lube, performing any of the strategies referred to above (especially jelqing) will be easier, more at ease and fun!

Natural oils work first-class and frequently include botanical, nutrition and antioxidant components. I propose you to choose these:

1.   Olive oil

2.   Almond oil

3.   Lavender oil

Just rub down these topically into your shaft, and they will enter through your pores and skin into deeper tissues!

Keep in mind: You'll discover quite a few lower priced lubricant oils on the market today, inclusive of VigRX Oil. So, before you strive any of these techniques, take into account to rub down your member

with a nutritious lube to achieve ideal
results.

#5. EAT ENOUGH PUMPKIN SEEDS

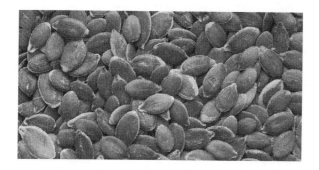

What many human beings don't realise is that total procedure of penis growth can be multiplied via a ideal weight loss plan (or supplements). By consuming proper you can extensively enhance the success you will have.

Pumpkin seeds have a LOT of strong vitamins that are acknowledged to make bigger and decorate blood waft and circulation, including:

1.

Phosphorou s – A nutrient that is acknowledged for presenting a wholesome libido. This is needed for anybody that has hassle getting it up.

2.   Zinc –

Testosterone is regulated partially via zinc.
This nutrient also approves for healthful
sperm manufacturing and ejaculation.
Zinc is necessary for the function of
testosterone and improvement of sperm.
The deficiency of zinc in men reasons
many sexual associated problems.

3.   Magnesium
– This nutrient is shown to enlarge blood
go with the flow and circulation in your
body. This is a mineral which plays an
essential position in producing intercourse
hormones like estrogen, androgen and and
other indispensable neurotransmitters.

4.   Selenium –
Approximately 50 percent of the selenium
in guys is current in seminal ducts and

testes. Men lose selenium in their semen & it is very vital to get adequate of this mineral for increased production and sperm condition.

As you can see, simply these three vitamins will have a large have an effect on on the excellent of your sex life. And, you'll also obtain an awful lot harder, higher looking erections in the process!

#6. TRY PENIS ENLARGEMENT HERBS

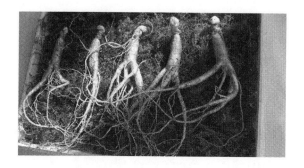

There are several herbs out there that can substantially enhance the blood glide into your penis. This way,your recuperation duration after doing workout routines will turn out to be an awful lot shorter and your outcomes a lot better.

Just focus on these herbs and components to improve your success rate:

- Korean crimson ginseng (improves blood drift and sexual features – be conscious that it contraindicates with a number of medications)

- Entengo herb (its properties are accountable for improving blood circulation in penis)

- Ginkgo biloba (improves sexual features if are suffering from anti-depressant-induced dysfunction – do now not take it if you are on blood thinners)

- Catuaba bark extract (highly environment friendly in augmenting sexual function, advertising deep relaxation, and improving your peripheral circulation)

- Maca powder (aphrodisiac that promotes better erectile feature and boosts electricity levels)

- Deer antler (it can draw extra blood to your penis for higher erections)

- Hawthorn berry (contains blood vessel strengthening dealers recognized as bioflavonoids)

- L-arginine (an amino acid that leads to multiplied blood waft – do now not take it if you are on nitroglycerin)

- Damiana (highly positive in addressing prostate troubles and impotence in males)

- Watermelon (contains an amino acid called citrulline, which gets transformed into arginine and leads to the dilation of blood vessels)

Most penis growth capsules have their formulas based on extracts from these flora and herbs. Just maintain in idea that these themselves will enhance only your blood flow. To acquire real size, you want to exercise.

#7. ERECTION BOOSTING ACTIVITIES YOU SHOULD DO

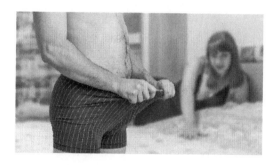

Guys, except all these pointers and tricks I have already furnished for you in this article, there are greater things you can do to improve your erections. I relatively propose you trying these things to do to enhance your size.

Lose weight from your belly:

Guys, this trick will no longer add to your size, but it will make you seem bigger. You recognize that stomach fat, specially all around your pelvis will cover phase of your shaft. The much less fats you will have, the more of your penis will be visible.

Trim down that pubic hair:

The pubic hair acts in a similar way as the belly fat. It hides part of your shaft. Therefore, I notably advise to at least trim it down (if now not absolutely shaving it). Once gone, your penis will now not solely seem to be greater hygienic and attractive, it will look even a little bit larger.

No pubic hair is something all female respect when giving you head. That ability you will get it greater often.

Avoid having laptop without delay on your lap:

Having a laptop computer on your lap is something you want to stop doing right now. The heat from this electric machine will reduce the quantity of your sperm remember and great of your erections.

Stop smoking:

Smoking is now not only hurting your body and health, it also hurts your sex life. Thanks to smoking, your bloodflow will be decreased and your penis will never attain its maximal erection potential.

Minimize your stress levels:

I bet you have already heard that the biggest erogenous zone in a man and a female is a brain. This organ triggers rush of a blood into your penis. When your brain is overstressed, then it has troubles to preserve appropriate erections. Therefore, try no longer to stress too an awful lot and meditate often.

Exercise regularly:

Except making you skinnier and searching great, working out and exercising (especially cardio workouts) will improve your bloodflow to the penis area. Not only that, it will raise your stamina and persistence that will enhance your sexual performance.

Sleep sufficient to recharge your penis:

Fred Joel

I wager you know about morning wood,
however did you be aware of that man can
have an erection at some stage in his sleep,
that can closing three to 5 hours? These
night-time boners convey blood into your
shaft to recharge and repair your penis –
keeping its desirable health.

#8. BOOST YOUR VITAMINS & MINERALS

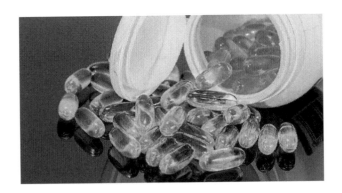

If you prefer to have more advantageous erections, better penis and more pleasurable intercourse life, you need to hold in mind your vitamins and minerals intake. Without desirable vitamins, your physique can't characteristic properly and you won't see the consequences you desire.

You need to focus on these vitamins & minerals to enhance your results:

Vitamins:

1. 2000 mg of Vitamin C twice or three instances a day

2. 30 mg of Zinc

3. 100 mg of Vitamin A

4. 200 mg of Magnesium

5. 100 IU of Vitamin D

6. 50 mg of Thiamine

Minerals that have a high-quality effect on sexual activity:

1. 525 mg of Calcium

2. 200 micrograms of Vitamin B12

3.   150 mg of Vitamin E

4.   25 micrograms of Potassium.

5.   400 micrograms of Folic Acid.

All of these minerals & vitamins can be discovered in your local pharmacy or on line in the shape of tablets or capsules.

CHAPTER 4

DIET TO ACHIEVE A
HEATHY PENIS

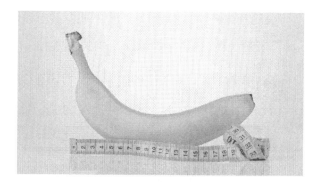

Did you understand that there are certain foods out there, that might help your penis health to thrive and prosper? In the subsequent few paragraphs, I will point out meals that can be offered in your nearby supermarket and won't cost you a fortune.

You need to center of attention on following:

•	Bananas – They are prosperous in potassium and also correct for your coronary heart and blood flow, bananas are honestly #1 endorsed meals for better penis fitness & intercourse life as well.

• Watermelon – Did you understand that watermelon is one of the few foods, that improve the size of your penis directly? Watermelon incorporates an amino acid referred to as citrulline, which is transformed to a popular amino acid that boosts health of your dick – arginine.

• Onions – Research shows that onions are superb for developing wholesome blood flow circulation for the duration of the body to the heart. Furthermore, onion consumption helps forestall blood clotting. But what humans seldom realise is that onions help not solely blood glide to the heart however additionally with blood flow to the penis.

• Salmon – Like we touched on in the case with onions, ingredients that generate a healthful blood glide are tested to assist you achieve stiffer erections. Eating salmon is no exception. Rich in Omega 3 and different fatty oils, salmon is great for thinning blood, which in turn helps generate a more healthy blood flow.

• Broccoli – You likely won't word any make bigger in penis girth or width, however broccoli is a remarkable vegetable for strengthening your pelvic muscles. If you don't like broccoli, attempt sweet potatoes, tomatoes, or even carrots.

• Low Fat Yogurt – Natural penis growth ingredients regularly incorporate excessive quantities of lean protein. Low-fat yogurt most really suits this as well as greek yogurt.

• Dark Chocolate – Dark chocolate contains flavonol, a phytochemical in a range of plant-based meals and beverages. What most human beings don't comprehend is that ingredients with flavonol, like darkish chocolate, are beneficial for growing blood waft to the penis. Plus dark chocolate tastes good!

SO GUYS, IF YOUR LITTLE BUDDY IS NOT PERFORMING AS IT USED TO BE, THEN IT'S THE BEST TIME TO START EATING THE RIGHT FOODS TO IMPROVE ITS FUNCTIONS!

CHAPTER 5

UNTOLD SECRETS OF ADDING MORE INCHES

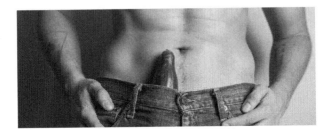

Well, the query is why shouldn't you? Doing penis workouts can raise not solely your length and girth but even the fitness of your penis (especially blood circulation and erection quality).

Keep in mind: As long as each you and your associate have a fulfilling sex lifestyles and are completely satisfied with the measurement or your manhood, there is no need to bear the prolonged method of "workout sessions".

It works on the identical principle as gaining new muscle when you work out in the gym. When exercising your muscle (or your penile tissue), you create microtears in your tissue.

Your physique then tries to fill in and restore these tearings and promotes cell boom in that area. This way, your muscle grows.

Pay attention: This identical principle is valid with regards to penis growth. There are even lookup research confirming that traction-based stretching can be permanent.

Luckily, the answer is sure – these workout routines are definitely safe as lengthy as you observe most important protection rules (as with any other workout program):

•   Starting gradual and steady is crucial.

•   Never pass warming up and warming down phases.

• You want to pay interest to the physiological procedures and warning signs your physique suggests to you (weak morning erections, soreness, red spots – all signs and symptoms you ought to no longer teach that hard).

Pay attention: If you have any fitness concerns, concerns or further questions, do not hesitate to talk with scientific professional earlier than you strive any new techniques.

If you overdo your education session, you can expect that some damage will happen. These are the most frequent ones:

– Spotting on the penis head, blisters, penis exhaustion, blood from penis, thrombosed vein, clogged lymph vessels, troubles with foreskin, penis no longer sensitive or overly sensitive, erectile dysfunction.

Keep in mind: Even when you work out in the fitness center and you are forcing your self too much, you can injure yourself. Working out your penis is the equal – overdo it and you are dealing with an injury.

Most guys ride one-inch growth in size and over a half-inch increase in girth surprisingly easily, however to be honest, you can get as massive as you want.

However, your effects and the speed at which you will reap your stop goals are man or woman and rely on following aspects:

- Workout regime you choose
- Dedication to routines you choose
- Your genetic capacity to cope with tissue changes

Keep in mind: You can locate a lot of guys on forums committed to dick expansion who gained lots more than the numbers I have cited above.

Luckily, your good points are permanent. Once you reach your favored size, you can stop your exercising regime (under some conditions). However, doing some light penis exercises is right to keep its appropriate health, erection excellent and growth.

Keep in mind: Once you reach your preferred dimension (phase one), you need to proceed with the 2d section during which you will make your positive factors permanent (also recognized as cementing your gains).

Guys, you want to realize that these manual exercises will now not deliver outcomes overnight because we are dealing with a day by day growth on a mobile basis. Therefore, achieving first visible good points will take round two to three weeks.

After that time, you must experience a great deal more impregnable erections while also you be able to study first dimension growth.

However, most guys report that the biggest increase they have experienced was once between the third and sixth month of constant and normal exercising. Pay attention: You will experience growth even after your sixth month, however, in addition good points will be a little bit slower.

Luckily, for a successful and permanent dimension gains, you do now not have to buy some thing as lengthy as you have two healthful hands. However, a number of equipment and devices dedicated to male enhancement will make the total process faster and a lot extra comfortable.

Here are the first-rate gadgets you can reflect onconsideration on getting your palms on:

- Hydro-based penis pumps (I propose Bathmate or Penomet) that will allow for a workout session while you take a bathe or bath.

- Penis extenders (my pinnacle three picks would be SizeGenetics, Male Edge or JesExtender, and Phallosan Forte) that will stretch your penis beneath your clothes whilst you do your every day activities.

Keep in mind: You can attain desirable consequences even besides these gadgets as long as you do exercises (explained in this article) manually & consistently. However, it will take you extra time and effort.

Sadly, an reply to this query is no longer a definitive YES or NO. Let me explain this a little bit more. There is no magic pill that will make your penis develop permanently on its own.

If you have problems with erection and bad blood glide into your penis, then you may also feel that after taking penis growth pills your penis has grown. In reality, you have only reached your maximum penis size thanks to more blood coming to your penis (because of accelerated blood flow).

However, many guys factor out the advantageous function of taking male enhancement drugs during your exercising session as a dietary assist for accomplishing even higher outcomes faster.

THE END

Made in the USA
Columbia, SC
11 May 2022

60272992R00046